YOUR KNOWLEDGE HAS VALUE

AF130111

- We will publish your bachelor's and master's thesis, essays and papers

- Your own eBook and book - sold worldwide in all relevant shops

- Earn money with each sale

Upload your text at www.GRIN.com and publish for free

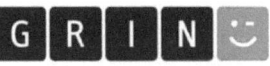

Bibliographic information published by the German National Library:

The German National Library lists this publication in the National Bibliography; detailed bibliographic data are available on the Internet at http://dnb.dnb.de .

Imprint:

Copyright © 2018 GRIN Verlag
Print and binding: Books on Demand GmbH, Norderstedt Germany
ISBN: 9783668755130

This book at GRIN:

https://www.grin.com/document/433599

Lameck Luwanda

Outbreak of Legionnaires' disease at the American Legion convention in Philadelphia in 1976

Current public health approaches to the prevention of further outbreaks

GRIN Verlag

GRIN - Your knowledge has value

Since its foundation in 1998, GRIN has specialized in publishing academic texts by students, college teachers and other academics as e-book and printed book. The website www.grin.com is an ideal platform for presenting term papers, final papers, scientific essays, dissertations and specialist books.

Visit us on the internet:

http://www.grin.com/

http://www.facebook.com/grincom

http://www.twitter.com/grin_com

A summary of an outbreak of Legionnaires' disease at the American Legion convention in Philadelphia in 1976 and its investigation: current public health approaches to the prevention of further outbreaks.

Table of contents:

1. Introduction

Legionnaires disease (LD) is a bacterial pneumonia dated back to the mid of 20th century. Its name came from the fact that it was first described within the legionnaires in Philadelphia, United States of America (USA) in the 1970s(1,2). It is a debilitating infection and causes many complications which, if not taken care of, are lethal. The causative bacteria are called *Legionella pneumophila;* they are also associated with a non-pneumonic form called Pontiac disease.

LD is thought to be transmitted through a mist of aerosols from contaminated water sources like respiratory therapy equipment, showers, decorative fountains, cooling systems, potting soil, humidifiers, and ice machines(3). The bacteria replicate in the water, and the vulnerable individual gets infected by inhaling the small water droplets called aerosols which get into the body through respiratory tract. The vulnerable individuals have been identified to be those with weakened immune system like smokers, alcohol abusers, cancer patients, patients with final stage renal disease and diabetes mellitus, advanced age, people living with human

1

immunodeficiency virus (HIV) or acquired immunodeficiency syndrome (AIDS) and those receiving drugs which suppress the immune system like steroids(3).

Epidemiologically, LD occurs worldwide mostly in the form of outbreaks and its diagnosis depends on the availability and capacity of the laboratories to perform a correct diagnosis. It is well diagnosed in developed countries due to the availability of resources. Bacterial culture is the gold standard, but there are also rapid serologic diagnostic tests which will be mentioned later in this easy.

The incidence varies worldwide, and this is due to the strength of surveillance and reporting systems. In the state of New York, the incidence trend has been reported to be increasing every year as seen in figure 1, and death rates are as high as 13% in treated patients(4). World Health Organization, WHO (5) reports that in the USA, Europe, and Australia there are approximately 10–15 cases detected per million.

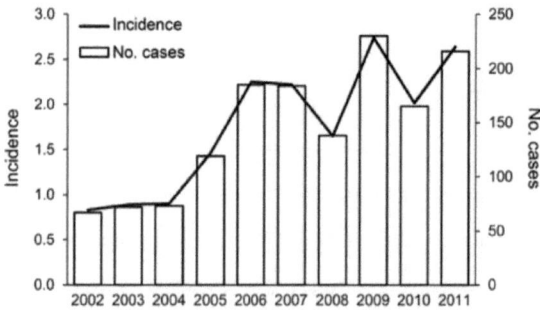

Figure 1: Annual number and incidence (no. cases/100,000 population) of Legionnaires' disease cases, New York, New York, USA, 2002–2011. Source: Farnham A, et al. Legionnaires' disease Incidence and Risk Factors, New York, USA, 2002–2011. Emerg Infect Dis, 2014; 20(11):1795-1802.

Clinically, LD has typically an incubation period of 2 to 10 days (1, 3, 4, 6) and modeling of LD outbreaks support an incubation period of six to seven days (7). The early symptoms include fever, loss of appetite, headache, malaise, and lethargy. A few patients may report muscle pain and confusion. There is usually a mild non-productive cough at the beginning; some patients develop phlegm. Progress to severe pneumonia and multiple organ failure occurs if no treatment is administered.

In this essay, description of the first reported outbreak of LD in the USA will be given followed by challenges and lessons learned until recently. Then, briefly, there will be a mention of current LD diagnostics tools and current methods used for public prevention.

2. The first Legionnaires' disease outbreak in the USA.

The first significant outbreak of LD occurred in summer of 1976 in Philadelphia, the USA among people who attended the 58th annual convention of the American Legion of the state of Pennsylvania(1). Official activities took place in the Bellevue-Stratford Hotel, and there was also another convention of the American Legion Auxiliary conducted in another hotel at the same time. Prior to1976, there were several pneumonia outbreaks resistant to penicillin in which the causative agent was not known with similar features, but currently, they are believed to have been caused by *Legionella pneumophila* (8). This microorganism was isolated and identified from lung tissues of dead patients to be a thin-walled gram-negative bacilli bacterium (2).

In the outbreak investigation, both clinical and epidemiological criteria were considered. Clinically a patient was supposed to have a fever, $38.5^{\circ}C$ or higher and cough or any fever with chest x-ray abnormality with onset between 1st of July and 18th of August. Epidemiologically the case was supposed to have been in the convention from 21st to 24th of July 1976 or to have entered the hotel. Those cases with only clinical criteria were termed to have "*broad street pneumonia.*"

Active case findings consisted of the search for patients in hospitals using public health trained nurses, and passively, a telephone hotline was set up so that the public could report any suspected case. Various surveys were conducted including hotel-guest surveys in four hotels to assess the rate at which the cases were meeting the clinical criteria, hotel-employee surveys to determine if they were affected by the disease, roommate surveys, hospital surveys in three hospitals to determine if the cases meeting the clinical criteria were occurring in other places apart from the convention and the Bellevue-Stratford Hotel, surveys of reported deaths due to pneumonia and influenza among Philadelphia residents from June to September of 1974, 1975 and 1976 and legionnaires survey questionnaires. Two more

3

case-control surveys were conducted. Samples were collected from the hotel environment, workers, and patients.

The entire outbreak included 182 patients who met clinical and epidemiological criteria. Of those, 82% attended the convention, and about 81% were hospitalized with a case fatality rate of 16% (1). The clinical features were similar to those described in the introduction. Half of those who died presented shock, and a majority kidney malfunction. From the record of 94 hospitalized patients, more than half presented leucocytosis, i.e., increased white blood cells. Chest radiographs were abnormal in 90% of hospitalized cases. The attack rate was found to increase with age, similar to what has been found in other outbreaks (4). Case fatality among those who met criteria for broad street pneumonia was 13%. The epidemic curve (Figure 2) showed a rapid increase soon after the start of the convention, then a plateau followed by a rapid decline of cases

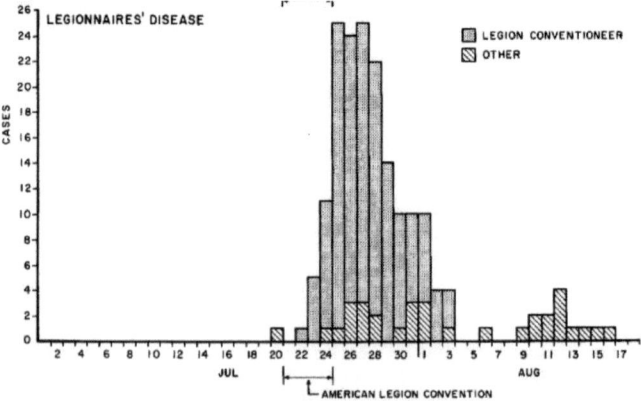

Figure 2: Epidemic curve of LD outbreak in 1976, Philadelphia. Source: Fraser, D.W. et al. Legionnaires' disease. Description of an epidemic of pneumonia. *N Engl J Med*. 1977; 297:1189-97.

The incubation period ranged from 2 to 10 days the except for two patients. The analysis showed that the Bellevue-Stratford Hotel was the primary site of exposure. It is also arguable that the causative agent was in the hotel for a long time because serologic tests found a higher proportion of titers in those who started to work before 1975. No association was found between LD and food or ice drinks served, but there was a significant association with drinking water at the hotel in those who met case definitions. Airborne transmission could not be proven but it was suspected as in other similar outbreak investigations (9,10).

3. Challenges and lessons learned since LD epidemic of 1976.

The 1976 LD outbreak in Philadelphia had challenges which helped the field of legionellosis to evolve and has increased the capability of health authorities to prevent it. I will discuss the challenges encountered in this first outbreak and others, and some of the lessons acquired and their incorporation into the new guidelines for public health prevention.

The primary challenge in the 1976 LD outbreak was *to figure out the type of microbe* that caused the disease. It costed a lot concerning resources and time, to discover that the cause was bacillus bacteria (2). Many tests had to be performed to rule out all known common pathogens. The presence of high fever could indicate the possibility of bacteria, but other pathogens like protozoa could also have caused high body temperature. Since the organism was not known, it was also a challenge to select the correct treatment. Various antibiotics were tried, but the results were generally poor except for those who were given erythromycin or tetracycline (1). Erythromycin belongs to the group of antibiotics called macrolide which forms the basis of current empirical treatment of LD (11-13). However, legionella species are currently showing resistance to macrolides (14), and therefore it is critical to test for legionella before administering antibiotics. The art of testing before treating may reduce the spread of resistance.

Failure to show the *mode of transmission* was another challenge in this outbreak, but there were some signs that airborne transmission could be the possible route(1). Eventually, it was discovered that a person could be infected when she inhales aerosols containing the bacteria (3). Many outbreaks have occurred in other parts of the world which also have confirmed that the disease is mainly air-borne and the bacteria lives in water with moderate temperature (3, 15). It is now well known that Legionella has many species and *L. pneumophila* is the most common and is associated with many cases of community-acquired (16, 17) and hospital-acquired pneumonia (6, 18).

5

Currently, there are guidelines for management of each disease including those occurring in epidemics like LD. Public Health of England (PHE), as well as the Centre for Disease Control (CDC) in the USA, have particular guidelines for LD control. These guidelines have evolved. The changes on these guidelines are due to new challenges realized from every known outbreak. Some of these challenges are preventable and may have played a role in the ascent of LD outbreaks in the USA as figure 3 displays (19). This surge in outbreaks in the USA prompted the public health authorities to implement the new guidance in 2015 for water system management (20).

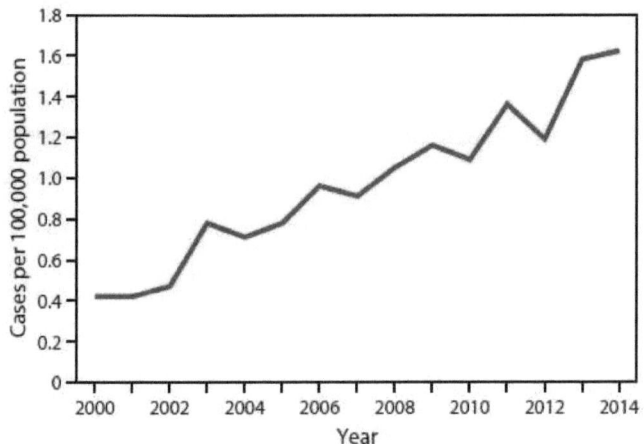

Figure 3: Reported cases of legionellosis per 100,000 population, by year — the United States, 2000–2014. Source: MMWR 2016.

For the United Kingdom, a rural LD outbreak in Hereford (21) in 2003 was a big lesson for the understanding of PHE. Hereford was not prepared for such a massive outbreak. Kirrage et al. (22) narrate that there was no office to act as an incident center, staff members were few and, as a result, each one had to undertake several duties at a time. Additionally, there were no explicit descriptions of roles and responsibilities. It has also been ascertained that flexibility in assuming different charges during an outbreak when there is a shortage of staff helps to ensure the flow of all control activities. One nursing manager said in an interview after the most significant LD outbreak in Furness General Hospital, Cumbria (23):

'It got to probably 4.35 pm or so and I thought to myself this place is absolutely heaving ... and I thought oh-oh—nights! We only have one night sister on duty at night ... so I checked with the Head of Nursing and said I should actually go home, sort a uniform out and come back in and work with the night sister. ... from then on I just worked night duty through to a week on Saturday'.

All challenges from the outbreaks have been taken into consideration by the PHE to make a clear guideline (24) for the control and management of legionellosis in England and Wales.

To simplify management and control of the LD outbreak, the CDC and PHE have devised three categories: travel associated, community and hospital acquired. Travel associated LD outbreaks are those occurring in accommodation sites, cruise ships and campsites. Community-acquired LD is caused by a common point source in the community, such as a contaminated water system. The hospital-acquired LD outbreak (HALD) occurs mostly when people get infected after being admitted to the hospital for two to ten days or having visited the source hospital in the last two to ten days. This definition of HALD has led to a suggestion by Francois Watkins et al. (25) that anyone who develops pneumonia after being admitted for two days in the hospital should be tested for LD. There is another category called healthcare-related outbreak which is associated with places like elderly care houses, and in practice, they are considered the same as community-acquired outbreaks.

Due to the nature of globalization and the possibility of spread, travel-associated LD outbreaks (TALD) have promoted cooperation among nations for proper control. For instance, the European Working Group for Legionella Infections (EWGLI) was founded in 1986 with the purpose of improving knowledge and information on epidemiological and microbiological aspects of LD. It interplays in forming regional guidelines for control and has a surveillance scheme called the European Legionnaires' Disease Surveillance Network (ELDSNet) since 1987 for tracking clusters, cases, and epidemics of LD (26). The data is also collected by the European Centre for Disease Prevention and Control (ECDC), which gather information through diseases-specific networks, and makes the information available to the public. The combination of these efforts has led to demonstrate that the information

7

about LD is underreported in Europe and there has been a rise in a number of LD outbreaks as figure 4 reveals (27). Eventually, when policymakers are aware of the gaps in identifying outbreaks, they will be in a position to form policies to enhance surveillance and thus reduce the chance of transmission and death within European territory.

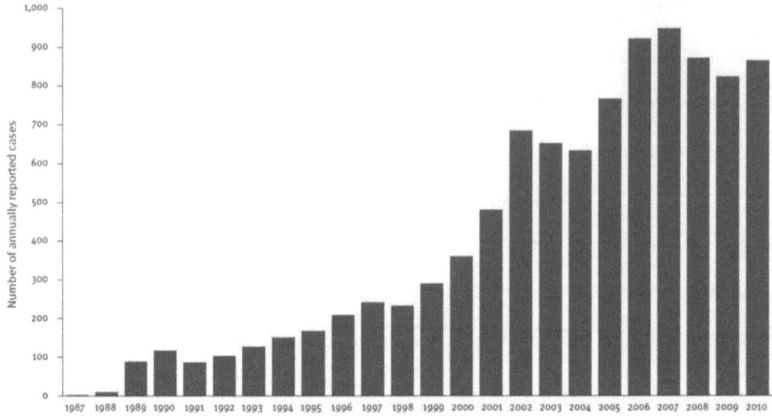

Figure 4: Annual number of reported cases of travel-associated Legionnaires' disease, EU/EEA countries, 1987–2010. Source: European Centre for Disease Prevention and Control (ECDC). Legionnaires' disease in Europe, 2010. Stockholm: ECDC; 2012.

Another challenge faced by the world is the lack of data of LD outbreaks from the African continent, especially sub-Saharan Africa (SSA). Lack of data of LD in SSA could be explained by a lack of proper investigation tools and weak health care systems which are not well established to conduct regular surveys. Still, there is a possibility of the presence of L.pneumophila because there is a high prevalence of community-acquired pneumonia and Legionella is one in the list of common causative agents (28). Nevertheless, after three years of the first description of LD epidemic in Philadelphia (USA), Kaplan et al. (29) started to report sporadic cases of LD in Johannesburg, and after that, there have been a couple of reports in hospital settings and immunocompromised patients in the South African Republic (30,31). South Africa is the only country in SSA that has reported LD cases. Due to lack of proper diagnostic tools in SSA, empirical treatment is deployed whenever LD is suspected. If this practice is sustained, allegedly, it will cause a surge in death rates due to antimicrobacterial resistance (AMR), if it is not happening already. It is also increasing the hospital costs for the patients.

4. Current advances in the diagnosis of LD

There are currently many diagnostic tests options for LD. Table 1 below provides the summary of tests available. Each of the methods has advantages and disadvantages, but in the scenario of LD suspicion, they can be used to complement each other. The gold standard continues to be a culture of the sputum, or blood samples (33, 34) and the rapid tests can easily be used to make a quick decision about the administration of correct antibiotics.

Test	Turnaround time	Sample type	Sensitivity, %	Specificity, %	Comments
Culture	3–7 Days	LRT	<10–80	100	Detects all species and serogroups
		Blood	<10	100	Too insensitive for clinical use
Direct fluorescent antibody staining	<4 h	LRT	25–70	>95	Technically demanding
Antigen detection	<1 h	Urine	70–90	>99	Only reliable for detection of *Legionella pneumophila* serogroup 1
Serological testing	3–10 Weeks	Serum	60–80	>95	Must test both acute- and convalescent-phase serum samples; single titer results can be misleading
PCR	<4 h	LRT	80–100	>90	No commercially available assay for testing clinical samples; detects all species and serogroups
		Serum	30–50	>90	—
		Urine	46–86	>90	—

NOTE. LRT, lower respiratory tract.

Table 1: Current diagnostic tests for legionnaires' disease. Source: Murdoch, D.R. (2003). Diagnosis of Legionella Infection *Clinical Infectious Diseases, 36,* 64–69

5. Current methods for public prevention

Methods which are currently used in the prevention of LD outbreaks can be summarized into three groups: methods to prevent the occurrence or spread of LD epidemics in hospitals, in the community, and among travelers. I will briefly discuss these methods separately below.

5.1 Prevention of LD hospital outbreak

First, it is necessary that all hospitals must follow guidelines provided by public health authorities. The guidelines have been simplified and are easy to use. Failure to follow them can increase the rates of LD epidemics as it has been reported in the US by Garrison et al. (19).

The most common way people are infected in hospital settings is through drinking water from the existing supplying system. Therefore, routine cultures of hospital drinking water samples can save lives. Some regular check-ups have shown that many hospitals have *L. pneumophila*, mostly serotype 1 which has been the cause of most outbreaks (35). The presence of the bacteria in the water sample can alert the physicians to consider possible etiology whenever they have a case of hospital-acquired pneumonia. On the other hand, it will potentially escalate the number of people treated empirically thus increasing the possibility of having AMR in the settings. Many US states and European countries have adopted the guidelines for regular environmental sampling and early detection of Legionella species according to Parr et al. (36) and Ricketts et al. (37). This adoption has already shown benefit in preventing the epidemic in hospitals in the Netherlands (38).

The second method to prevent LD outbreaks in the hospital is to disinfect water supply sources. There are many techniques used for this particular purpose. Hyperchlorination was the first technique which consisted of raising the concentration of chlorine to the maximum in the water supply for 24 hours. After those many setbacks were observed. In a study (39) conducted in a hospital in Italy, hyperchlorination showed to be effective at the beginning, but after two months the levels of Legionella species increased as shown in figure 5. Hyperchlorination also reduces the water quality if chlorine is sustained at a high level to kill the microorganisms (40). Therefore, it is currently not preferred.

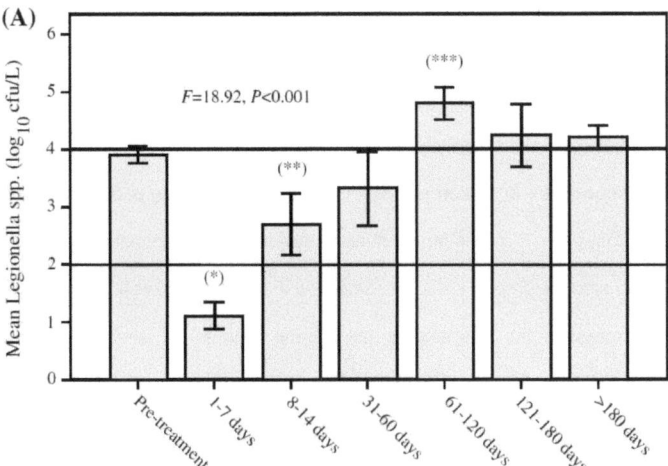

(A)

Figure 5: Concentration of legionella colonies with hyperchlorination as observed with time. Source: Marchesi, I., Marchegiano, P., Bargellini, A. et al. Effectiveness of different methods to control Legionella in the water supply: ten-year experience in an Italian university hospital. *Journal of Hospital Infection, 2010; 77(1):47-51.*

Another technique to disinfect water is *superheating-and-flush*. It consists of raising the water temperature very high above 60^0C and flushing it out. The bacteria cannot survive under high temperature. Lin et al. (41) have suggested that this technique should be used as an emergency during an epidemic in the hospital with or without hyperchlorination.

Thirdly, the use of *chlorine dioxide* is another effective disinfection method for preventing LD outbreak in hospital settings. Chlorine dioxide is a potent oxidant agent produced by electrolysis and is capable of inhibiting or killing the microbes (42, 43). Ma et al. (44) have demonstrated that it has a high antimicrobial activity of over 98% and several studies (45-48) have shown that it is inexpensive. All by-products formed during the electrical activity are at low concentration and safe for human use. It is the best technique due to low chances of having harmful health effects and value for money.

Finally, installation of *copper-silver ionization units* has shown positive results in preventing LD outbreaks. It also consists of producing ions through electrolysis which kill the microbes. One study (49) has reported that the first sixteen hospitals to deploy this technique have not reported any case of LD for more than ten years. This particular technique has been the only one to fulfill all four scientific evaluation criteria among all disinfection modalities.

5.2. Prevention of LD epidemic in the community

The first measure to prevent an epidemic in the community is to create awareness. This awareness can be through education in the promotion and prevention specific programs or to include it in other campaigns against respiratory infections. However, if the magnitude of the problem is unknown, like in African settings, it is difficult to educate people because there is no concrete information. It is time for healthcare providers in African settings, like established HIV cohorts, to start looking for the *L. pneumophila* in patients with respiratory complications and those admitted in the hospitals. It will provide data to be used for advocating the challenge and formulate new health policies.

There are a few proven techniques for controlling LD outbreaks in the community. The best known is the application of *monochlaramine* in water systems. Monochloramine is a known disinfectant compound formed through a combination of hydrochlorous salt and ammonia. Several studies (50-53) have shown that if it is applied correctly in the municipal water supply systems, it can reduce colonization of *L. pneumophila* by 90%. It is also applied in the hospitals and widely used in the US and Europe for disinfecting large water supplies for the communities. When the monochloramine method is used together with chlorine dioxide, legionella colonies are entirely eliminated (54). Allegedly, for better control of the LD epidemic in our societies, we should combine these two methods.

5.3.   Prevention of travel associated LD outbreak.

Currently, there are no vaccines or prophylactic treatments for legionnaires' disease. People with known risk factors are advised to avoid high-risk areas like spas and pools. Also, local public health authorities should be quick to act whenever LD outbreak is detected in accommodation sites, cruises or campsites. A good example was the rapid response of Shelby County health officials, near Memphis International Airport, Tennessee to shut down The La Quinta Inn & Suites after being suspected to be the source of LD outbreak (55).

6. Conclusion

In this essay, I started with general information followed by the short description of the very first reported LD outbreak in the world, which occurred in Philadelphia, USA. The description gave a picture of how information was collected. The case fatality rate in this outbreak was 16% and the incubation period was determined to be 2 to 10 days. Subsequently, I discussed some of the challenges and lessons learned from this and subsequent LD outbreaks. The main challenges in the first outbreak were associated with the unknown nature of the causative agent regarding its type, treatment, and mode of transmission. I explained that the lessons learned have been used to formulate new guidelines and formation of regional cooperation like EWGLI which has helped to identify gaps in reporting. I have also highlighted the lack of LD information in sub-Saharan Africa and its importance. The diagnostics have been briefly discussed and culture remains to be the gold standard. Prevention methods have been discussed in three groups, namely, hospital, community, and travel associated preventions. In hospital prevention, a culture of the environmental sample has been shown to be very important, and the use of disinfection techniques are the most successful. For the community, a combination of monochloramine and chloride dioxide has the possibility of clearing all the legionella colonies when used in water systems.

Since 1976, public health authorities have learned and obtained experiences with the outbreaks. However, there is a need to strengthen the surveillance systems, as there has been an increase in the number of LD outbreaks. The day vaccine for LD would be available, especially for *L.pneumophila* serotype 1; people at high risk must be prioritised.

7. References.

1. Fraser DW, Tsai TR, Orenstein W, Parkin WE, Beecham HJ, Sharrar RG, et al. Legionnaires' disease. Description of an epidemic of pneumonia. *N Engl J Med.* 1977; 297(22): 1189-97.
2. McDade JE, Shepard CC, Fraser DW, Tsai TR, Redus MA, Dowdle WR. Legionnaires' disease. Isolation of a bacterium and demonstration of its role in other respiratory disease. *N Engl J Med.* 1977; 297(22):1197-1203
3. Woo AH, Goetz A, Yu VL. Transmission of Legionella by Respiratory Equipment and Aerosol Generating Devices. *Chest.*1992; 102(5):1586–1590. *Available at: http://dx.doi.org/10.1378/chest.102.5.1586*
4. Farnham A, Alleyne L, Cimini D, Balter S. Legionnaires' Disease Incidence and Risk Factors, New York, New York, USA, 2002–2011. *Emerg Infect Dis*, 2014; 20(11): 1795-1802. Available at: https://dx.doi.org/10.3201/eid2011.131872
5. World Health Organization. *Legionellosis.* Available from: http://www.who.int/mediacentre/factsheets/fs285/en/ [Accessed on 7th April 2017]
6. Kirby BD, Snyder KM, Meyer RD, Finegold SM. Legionnaires' disease: report of sixty-five nosocomially acquired cases of review of the literature. *Medicine (Baltimore).* 1980; 59:188.
7. Egan J, Hall I, Lemon D J, Leach SA. Modelling Legionnaires' disease outbreaks: estimating the timing of an aerosolized release using symptom-onset dates *Epidemiology.* 2011;22(2):188-98
8. Baine WB. Ill winds and troubled waters: selected whiffs of legionellosis. *Ann.Ist.Super.Sanità.* 1983;19(2-3):215-240
9. U.S Department of Health, Education and Welfare. *Institutional outbreak of pneumonia.* Morbid Mortal Weekly Report: 14:265-286, 1965.
10. U.S Department of Health, Education and Welfare. *Epidemic of obscure illness-Pontiac, Michigan.* Morbid Mortal Weekly Report: 17:315-320, 1968.
11. Miller, A.C. Erythromycin in legionnaires' disease: a re-appraisal. *J Antimicrob Chemother. 1981;* 7(3):217-22.
12. Vergis EN, Indorf A, et al. Azithromycin vs cefuroxime plus erythromycin for empirical treatment of community-acquired pneumonia in hospitalized patients: a prospective, randomized, multicenter trial. *Arch Intern Med.* 2000; 160:1294.
13. Fraser DW, Wachsmuth I, Bopp C, et al. Antibiotic treatment of guinea-pigs infected with agent of Legionnaires' disease. *Lancet*, 1978; 1:175.
14. Sikora A, Gładysz I, Kozioł-Montewka M, et al. Assessment of antibiotic susceptibility of Legionella pneumophila isolated from water systems in Poland. *Ann Agric Environ Med*, 2017; 24(1):66-69. Available at: doi: 10.5604/12321966.1234048.
15. Tabatabaei M, Hemati Z, Moezzi M, Azimzadeh N. Isolation and identification of *Legionella* spp. from different aquatic sources in south-west of Iran by molecular & culture methods. *Molecular Biology Research Communications.* 2016; 5(4):215–223.
16. Marrie TJ, Peeling RW, Fine MJ, et al. Ambulatory patients with community-acquired pneumonia: the frequency of atypical agents and clinical course. *Am J Med.*1996; 101: 508.
17. Fang GD, Fine M, Orloff J, et al. New and emerging etiologies for community-acquired pneumonia with implications for therapy. A prospective multicenter study of 359 cases. *Medicine (Baltimore).* 1990; 69,307.
18. Sabria M, Yu VL. Hospital-acquired legionellosis: solutions for a preventable infection. *Lancet Infect Dis,* 2002; 2(6):368-73.
19. Garrison LE, Kunz JM, Cooley LA. *Deficiencies in Environmental Control Identified in Outbreaks of Legionnaires' Disease — North America, 2000–2014.* Morbidity and Mortality Weekly Report: 65(22)
20. ASHRAE. ASHRAE 188-2015. *Legionellosis: Risk Management for Building Water Systems.* New York: McGraw-Hill;2015

21. Kirrage D, Reynolds G, Smith GE, et al. Investigation of an outbreak of Legionnaires' disease: Hereford, UK 2003. *Respir Med, 2007;* 101(8):1639-44.
22. Kirrage D, Hunt D, Ibbotson S, et al. Lessons learned from handling a large rural outbreak of Legionnaires' disease: Hereford, UK 2003. *Respir Med.* 2007; 101(8): 1645–1651. Available at: http://doi.org/10.1016/j.rmed.2007.03.010
23. Smith AF, Wild C, Law J. The Barrow-in-Furness legionnaires' outbreak: qualitative study of the hospital response and the role of the major incident plan. *Emerg Med J,* 2005; 22(4): 251-5. Available at: DOI:10.1136/emj.2004.014316
24. Public Health England. *Guidance on investigating cases, clusters and outbreaks of Legionnaires' disease.* London: Crown;2016
25. Francois Watkins LKF, Toews K, Harris AM, et al. Lessons From an Outbreak of Legionnaires' Disease on a Hematology-Oncology Unit. *Infect Control Hosp Epidemiol.2017;* 38:306-313. Available at: DOI: 10.1017/ice.2016.281
26. Hutchinson EJ, Joseph CA, Bartlett CL. EWGLI: a European surveillance scheme for travel associated legionnaires' disease. *Eurosurveillance.* 1996;1 (5):37–39
27. European Centre for Disease Prevention and Control. Legionnaires disease in Europe, 2010. Stockholm: ECDC; 2012.
28. Feldman C, Brink AJ, Richards GA, Maartens G, Bateman ED. Management of community-acquired pneumonia in adults. *South African Medical Journal,* 2007; 97(12): 1296–1306.
29. Kaplan C, Zwi S, Kallenbach J, et al. Legionnaires' disease in Johannesburg. *S Afr Med J,* 1980; 58(1):13-7.
30. Strebel PM, Ramos JM, Eidelman IJ, et al. Legionnaires' disease in a Johannesburg teaching hospital. Investigation and control of an outbreak. *S Afr Med J,* 1988; 73(6): 329-33.
31. Wolter N, Carrim M, Cohen C, et al. Legionnaires' Disease in South Africa, 2012– 2014. *Emerging Infectious Diseases,* 2016; 22(1):131-133. Available at: https://dx.doi.org/10.3201/eid2201.150972.
32. Murdoch DR. Diagnosis of Legionella Infection *Clinical Infectious Diseases, 2003;*36:64–9
33. Fields BS, Benson RF, Besser RE. *Legionella* and Legionnaires' disease: 25 years of investigation. *Clin Microbiol Rev* 2002; 15:506–526. Available at: http://dx.doi.org/10.1128/CMR.15.3.506-526.2002.
34. Heuner K, Swanson M. *Legionella: molecular microbiology.* Norfolk: Caister Academic Press;2008
35. Stout JE, Muder RR, Mietzner S, et al. Role of environmental surveillance in determining the risk of hospital-acquired legionellosis: a national surveillance study with clinical correlations. *Infect Control Hosp Epidemiol,* 2007;28:818-24. Available at: DOI: https://doi.org/10.1086/518754
36. Parr A, Whitney EA, Berkelman RL. Legionellosis on the Rise: A Review of Guidelines for Prevention in the United States. *Journal of Public Health Management and Practice,* 2015; 21(5): E17-E26. Available at: doi:10.1097/PHH.0000000000000123.
37. Ricketts KD, Joseph CA. The impact of new guidelines in Europe for the control and prevention of travel-associated Legionnaires' disease. *Int. J. Hyg. Environ.-Health,* 2006; 209:547–552. Available at: doi:10.1016/j.ijheh.2006.05.003
38. Den Boer JW, Verhoef L, Bencini MA, et al. Outbreak detection and secondary prevention of Legionnaires' disease: A national approach. *Int. J. Hyg. Environ.-Health,* 2006;210:1–7 Available at: doi:10.1016/j.ijheh.2006.07.00
39. Marchesi I, Marchegiano P, Bargellini A, et al. Effectiveness of different methods to control legionella in the water supply: ten-year experience in an Italian university hospital. *Journal of Hospital Infection,* 2010; 77(1):47-51. Available at: oi:10.1016/j.jhin.2010.09.012
40. Orsi GB, Vitali M, Marinelli L, Ciorba V, Tufi D,Del Cimmuto A, et al. Legionella control in the water system of antiquated hospital buildings by shock and continuous

hyperchlorination: 5 years experience. *BMC Infectious Diseases,* 2014;14:394 Available at: DOI: 10.1186/1471-2334-14-394
41. Lin YE, Stout JE, Yu VL. Controlling Legionella in hospital drinking water: an evidence-based review of disinfection methods. *Infect Control Hosp Epidemiol,* 2011; 32(2):166-73. Available at: doi: 10.1086/657934.
42. Sanekata T, Fukuda T, Miura T, et al. Evaluation of the antiviral activity of chlorine dioxide and sodium hypochlorite against feline calicivirus, human influenza virus, measles virus, canine distemper virus, human herpesvirus, human adenovirus, canine adenovirus and canine parvovirus. *Biocontrol Sci.* 2010; 15:45–49. Available at: doi: 10.4265/bio.15.45
43. Ogata N, Shibata T. Protective effect of low-concentration chlorine dioxide gas against influenza a virus infection. *J. Gen. Virol. 2008;* 89: 60–67. Available at: doi: 10.1099/vir.0.83393-0
44. Ma JW, Huang BS, Hsu CW, et al. Efficacy and Safety Evaluation of a Chlorine Dioxide Solution. *International Journal of Environmental Research and Public Health.* 2017; *14*(3): 329. Available at: http://doi.org/10.3390/ijerph14030329
45. Srinivasan A, Bova G, Ross T, et al. A 17-Month Evaluation of a Chlorine Dioxide Water Treatment System to Control Legionella Species in a Hospital Water Supply. *Infection Control & Hospital Epidemiology,* 2003; 24(8): 575-579. Available at: doi:10.1086/502254
46. Zhang Z, McCann C, Stout J, et al. Safety and Efficacy of Chlorine Dioxide for Legionella Control in a Hospital Water System. *Infection Control & Hospital Epidemiology.* 2007; *28*(8):1009-1012. Available at: doi:10.1086/518847
47. Marchesi I, Marchegiano P, Bargellini A, et al. Effectiveness of different methods to control legionella in the water supply: ten-year experience in an Italian university hospital. *Journal of Hospital Infection.* 2010; 77(1):47-51 Available at: oi:10.1016/j.jhin.2010.09.012.
48. Zhang Z, McCann C, Hanrahan J, et al. Legionella control by chlorine dioxide in hospital water systems. *American Water Works Association Journal.* 2009; 101(5):117-127,   12.   Retrieved   from https://search.proquest.com/docview/221595862?accountid=13042
49. Stout JE, Yu VL. Experiences of the First 16 Hospitals Using Copper-Silver Ionization for Legionella Control: Implications for the Evaluation of Other Disinfection Modalities. *Infection Control and Hospital Epidemiology.* 2015;24(8):563-568 Available at: DOI: https://doi.org/10.1086/502251
50. Flannery B, Gelling LB, Vugia DJ, et al. Reducing Legionella colonization in water systems with monochloramine. *Emerg Infect Dis, 2006;* 12:588.
51. Weinraub JM, Flannery B, Vugia DJ, Gelling LB, Salerno JJ, Stevens VA, et al. Legionella' Reduction after Conversion to Monochloramine for Residual Disinfection. *Journal (American Water Works Association).* 2008; 100(4): 129–139. Retrieved from http://www.jstor.org/stable/41314606
52. Moore MR, Pryor M, Fields B, et al. Introduction of Monochloramine into a Municipal Water System: Impact on Colonization of Buildings by *Legionella* spp. *Appl. Environ. Microbiol.* 2005; 72(1):378-38. Available at: doi: 10.1128/AEM.72.1.378-383.2006
53. Melada S, Coniglio MA. Monochloramine for Remediation of Legionella Only in Domestic Hot Water Systems: An Iron Fist in a Velvet Glove. *Open Journal of Preventive   Medicine.   2015;   5:   143-150.   Available   at:* http://dx.doi.org/10.4236/ojpm.2015.53017
54. Marchesi I, Ferranti G, Bargellini A, et al. Monochloramine and Chlorine Dioxide for Controlling Legionella pneumophila Contamination: Biocide Levels and Disinfection By-Product Formation in Hospital Water Networks. *Journal of Water and Health.* 2013; 11:738-747. Available at: http://dx.doi.org/10.2166/wh.2013.079
55. Charlier T. *Memphis hotel shut down after outbreak of Legionnaires' Disease confirmed.* Available from:

http://archive.commercialappeal.com/news/government/county/memphis-hotel-shut-down-after-outbreak-of-legionnaires-disease-confirmed-3d1a0af3-b5eb-4c85-e053-010-394426961.html [Accessed on 8th April 2017]

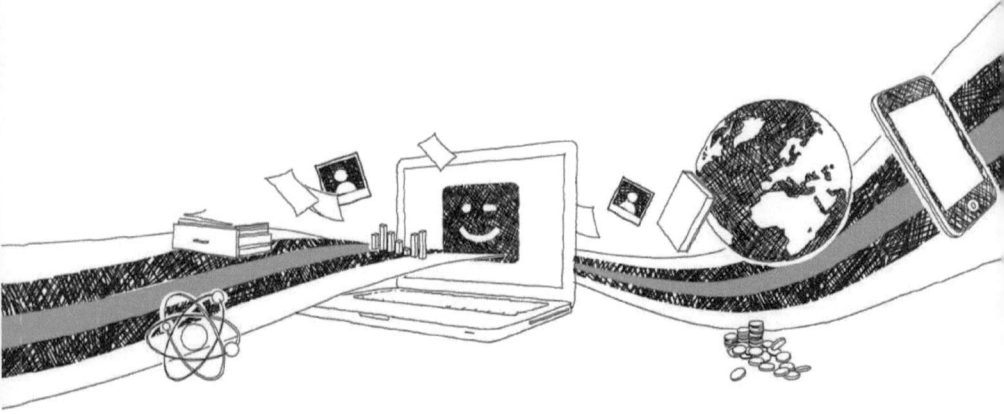
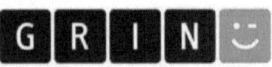